A GUIDE TO NON-SURGICAL AESTHETICS

The Steps Necessary To Make YOU
Beautiful On The Outside

KEVIN COUGHLIN
DMD, MBA, MAGD, L.E.

Foreword

I want to say thank you to my wife, Karen, and three children who continue to support my decisions no matter how crazy they seem!

To my brother, Dr. Bret Coughlin, for his knowledge, love of medicine, and his desire to always do what is right.

I want to thank the Ochoa Family, Margaret, Myles, Troy, and Zoey. Thank you to their business, Ochoa Salon and Spa, that shares in my passion to provide clients with the best service, knowledge, and education to help clients achieve the best esthetic results.

To Mr. Bill Ochoa whose passion for life and love of cosmetics opened the door in the field of aesthetics with the idea of making you beautiful on the outside while making you feel beautiful on the inside.

About the Author

Dr. Coughlin is a practicing dentist, with a focus on cosmetics since 1983. Dr. Coughlin holds a master's in healthcare administration, a master's in the academy of general dentistry, and a license as an esthetician. Kevin, along with his brother Dr. Bret Coughlin and the Ochoa family, decided that it was time to provide guidance, knowledge, and information to their most important asset, their clients and patients, to help them make intelligent and well-informed decisions when it comes to non-surgical aesthetics. We believe this guide is one of the many steps to achieve this goal.

Table of Contents

Preface

During the practice of non-surgical aesthetics, it became clear that one of the most important aspects in helping clients achieve their goal of external beauty is to help clients understand what can and cannot be achieved through non-surgical options. For this reason, I designed a book that would answer these basic questions. It is important for clients to become as informed as possible before undergoing a non surgical procedure or for that matter any procedure. I want to provide clients with the information to become better informed before receiving or deciding upon a treatment. Although no guide can completely answer every question when it comes to the rapidly changing field of cosmetics, this guide is sought to provide information that will make your consultation visit more valuable. My goal is to help better inform you so you can obtain the best results in the most comprehensive fashion using the latest techniques.

CHAPTER 1

What is Beauty?

Beauty means many things to many different people. In this context however, the goal of beauty is a focus on external physical beauty and our ability to offer products and services to help achieve results that improve the tone, texture, and tightness to the largest organ of the body, your skin. As the client, your job is to make yourself beautiful on the inside. One way to help accomplish internal beauty is feeling good about your body on the outside too.

For the best results, we must start by fully understanding what can and what cannot be achieved. The clinician, the aesthetician, and the client must be on the same page. The first step in accomplishing this is through transparent communication while establishing a common realistic goal.

In my opinion, expectations need to be defined from the start. For example, does the client want to achieve an artificial, an unnatural esthetic, or a natural more realistic result? Goals such as these need to be determined. I caution every client to consider minor changes to their skincare over long periods of time. These changes include emphasizing proven strategies to reduce damage to your skin and applying proven products and procedures. In doing so, you also need to maintain enough maturity to understand that we all age and are subject to mother nature. Our goal is to outsmart her as much as possible by minimizing the adverse effects of the aging process as for as long as possible.

The power of appearance and the force of image can have a tremendous impact on how we perceive ourselves and how others perceive us. True long-term beauty must start with overall health, which means a healthy lifestyle, healthy diet, and a healthy outlook on life! Please do not discount these pillars of beauty. We all know beautiful people that are miserable so please be aware that your long-term goals should include a healthy balance of intellect for your mind, exercise for your body, and faith for your soul.

In almost all cases beauty can be a universal language. For women, large eyes, high cheekbones, and full lips are generally seen as externally beautiful features. However, the human eye sees averages or blends that provide our brain with a subconscious idea of external beauty. Thus, the more your features are blended, the better the results. In substance, the combination of small eyes with big lips will tell our subconscious that our face is out of balance and the goal of attaining beauty can be lost.

To achieve facial beauty, you should consider all elements; the smile, the lip line, the smile line, the color of teeth, the shape of teeth, the shape of the face, the height of the cheekbones, the size of your eyes, the shape of your nose, the fullness of your lips, the shape of your chin, and the complexion of your skin along with the tone, texture, and color of your skin. Remember that balance and symmetry provide the best recipes for beauty.

CHAPTER 2

How Do You Attain Beauty?

You are making an investment in yourself; you are about to spend money and time to improve your appearance so consider the following. Most people have poor skin conditions because of their unhealthy lifestyle.

Roughly 85% of poor skin conditions occur because of sun damage. Think about it, 85%! So, what can you do? You do not necessarily have to avoid the sun you just must control your exposure to it. In general terms the sun has UVA, UVB, and UVC rays. UVA rays are the rays you are exposed too from tanning beds so remember this, the A in UVA should stand for aging since the more you use a tanning bed the more your skin will age. The B in UVB should stand for burning because the more B rays you are exposed to the more your skin burns. Lastly, the C in UVC should mean cancer because it is the C rays that change your cellular composition in your cells that cause one of the three main types of skin cancer. These three main types of skin cancer are Basal Cell, Squamous Cell, and Malignant Melanoma. As you can see, it is important to wear the appropriate sunscreen with a SPF of 40 or higher. It is also important to remember to purchase new sunscreen every season since the effectiveness does wear away and make sure you apply multiple times throughout the day. When purchasing sunscreen keep in mind it should contain between 8-10% zinc oxide and titanium dioxide.

So, what about the other 15%? This encompasses your genes, diet, and lifestyle. Let's start with your DNA. Some of you are just lucky, you have hit the jackpot and inherited great genes from your parents. The tone, texture, and tightness along with color of your skin is perfect so don't go and mess it up. Others will need to work harder to achieve impressive results. It can happen and you owe it to yourself to allow it to happen. Most clients will have dry, oily, normal, a combination of dry and oily, or sensitive skin. Your skin type should be identified and products should be applied daily or in some cases multiple times a day to help you win the battle against the elements that are causing your skin to prematurely age. The next target area is your diet. As many of you know this is no great surprise, you are what you eat. In my opinion, one habit to avoid above all others is stop smoking and consuming alcohol. We all know this most likely will not occur so it is important to consider moderation, such as no more than 1-2 cigarettes a day and no more than one to two ounces of alcohol a day. Also, try reducing or eliminating caffeine products, sugary beverages, and greasy saturated fats to help promote a good healthy diet. Although many times the last item lifestyle will get only lip service high stress, poor sleeping habits, and a toxic environment will certainly not only age your skin but also significantly contribute hypertension along with many other cardiovascular issues.

Clients should let clinicians and estheticians guide them through the vast array of products and services not only to get your skin healthy, but also keep it healthy.

CHAPTER 3

What is RF or Radio-Frequency?

RADIO FREQUENCY

What is Radio Frequency or RF? It is any of the electromagnetic wave frequencies that lie in the range extending from around 3 kHz to 300GHz. It is the range which includes those frequencies used for communication or radar signals. In most cases, RF usually refers to electrical rather than mechanical oscillations; however, mechanical RF systems do exist.

RF can heat up the skin and or surrounding nerve tissue to stimulate new collagen in the subdermal area to reduce the appearance of fine lines and loose skin and can be a first step to avoiding a surgical procedure such as a face lift. The goal in RF is to heat the skin to 40-42 degrees Centigrade or roughly 108 degrees Fahrenheit for a period of time to get the best results. Your external skin temperature will be monitored by another device to make sure we do not under or over heat your skin. The use of RF can be used on any part of your body. In most cases a procedure will take between 30-40 minutes. In most cases we will recommend starting with 2-4 treatments to get a jump start in making your skin look and feel the best. After this initial jump start period we will usually recommend maintenance treatments every 3-4 months. Once your treatments are completed you will have no down time and be able to put makeup on immediately and although we do not recommend sun exposure there is no direct contra-indication to sun exposure which makes RF convenient and easy for most clients.

WHO CAN BENEFIT FROM RF TREATMENT?

Clients who have mild to lax type skin are usually the best candidates for this type of treatment, and clients with thinner skin will have more success than those with thicker skin. Treatments with RF are most suitable for the brow area, the cheeks, nasolabial folds, jowls and neck area. RF treatment will also be effective on the treatment of rhytides or wrinkles, acne and cellulite reduction.

RF PROS AND CONS

RF is treatment that can give great results by tightening the skin and one of the only methods which has very little down time for are clients. What this means is less interference in your day to day activities. Discomfort is minimized by cool tip procedure; however, topical anesthesia can be used on more sensitive clients.

HOW RF IS PERFORMED?

In order to ensure that the treatment is even throughout the procedure, many times a grid will be drawn on the area to be treated. During the treatment you can expect to feel heat, cold and then heat again. It is important that you the client stay still during the procedure to prevent thermal injury to your skin. Each area or grid for treatment will last about two seconds and we will move to the next designated area. Each treatment will last between 30-60 minutes. Most clients treated with RF will notice immediate tightening of the skin however for optimal results treatment should be repeated until desired results are obtained. Most clients will notice mild swelling and redness with some lumpiness seen in the areas where the skin is thinner than others; most symptoms will subside over a few weeks. In some cases clients have mentioned itching, numbness and intermittent pain for as long as several months and this appears more common along the jawline and cheekbones.

RADIO FREQUENCY SKIN TIGHTENING PROCEDURES

On the day of your radio frequency skin tightening procedure you should avoid wearing any cosmetics or lotion, especially oil-based formulas, as they may affect how effectively the RF waves make contact with the skin. After you sit down, your provider will spread a numbing cream on your skin to decrease the chances of discomfort. After the cream has sufficiently numbed the skin, he or she will use a grid transfer to improve the precision of the radio frequency skin tightening procedure. The skin care specialist will then use a gliding gel to increase the effectiveness of the delivery to the skin in order to reduce the chances of irritation. If you have sensitive skin and feel any kind of heat sensation after the treatment, you can request a cooling mist or thin gel to reduce or eliminate these sensations.

RADIO FREQUENCY SKIN TIGHTENING SIDE EFFECTS

While radio frequency skin tightening has a lower instance of side effects than other cosmetic and non-invasive procedures, there are still several risks involved. Common side effects that have been reported include mild swelling of the treated skin, redness, sinking of the treated area, and sensitivity. You should monitor the treated skin carefully during the first few hours after treatment to ensure that your skin isn't reacting negatively to the treatment. Do not touch or manipulate the area too much, as this might cause further irritation. If the heated sensations return, you can use a spray bottle to mist the area with cool water and an Aloe Vera mixture. If you should experience severe swelling, pain, or other unusual side effects, you should call immediately, as these may be signs of a serious side effect to the radio frequency skin tightening treatment.

CHAPTER 4

What is IPL or Intense Pulsed Light?

Intense pulsed light (**IPL**) is a technology used by cosmetic and medical practitioners to perform various skin treatments for aesthetic and therapeutic purposes, including hair removal, photo rejuvenation (e.g. the treatment of skin pigmentation, sun damage, and thread veins) as well as to alleviate dermatologic diseases such as acne. IPL is increasingly used in ophthalmology as well, to treat evaporative dry eye disease due to Meibomian gland dysfunction.

The technology uses a high-powered, hand-held, computer-controlled flashgun to deliver an intense, visible, broad-spectrum pulse of light, generally in the visible spectral range of 400 to 1200 nm. Various cutoff filters are commonly used to selectively filter out lower wavelengths, especially potentially damaging ultraviolet light. The resulting light has a spectral range that targets specific structures and chromophores (e.g. melanin in hair, or oxyhemoglobin in blood vessels) that are heated to destruction and reabsorbed by the body. IPL shares some similarities with laser treatments, in that they both use light to heat and destroy their targets. But unlike lasers that use a single wavelength (color) of light which typically matches only one chromophore, and hence only one condition, IPL uses a broad spectrum that when used with filters, allows it to be used against several conditions. This can be achieved when the IPL technician selects the appropriate filter that matches a specific chromophore.

The first FDA approval of IPL was for telangiectasia in 1995. Use quickly spread to a variety of medical and cosmetic settings. Treatment is generally safe and effective, but complications can occur such as hyperpigmentation. The polychromatic light can reach multiple chromophores in human skin: mainly hemoglobin, water, and melanin. This results in selective photothermolysis of the target, which can be blood vessels, pigmented cells, or hair follicles.

Broad-spectrum light is applied to the surface of the skin, targeting melanin. This light travels through the skin until it strikes the hair shafts or the bulb (root). The bulb is usually where the highest concentration of melanin is located. As the light is absorbed, the bulb and most of the hair shaft are heated, destroying the hair-producing papilla.There are also claims that heat conversion occurs directly in the darker capillaries that bring blood to the follicle.

At any one time, not all hair follicles are active and only active hair follicles can be affected by the treatment. Inactive hair follicles can be treated as they become active over time. For IPL treatments, an average of 8–10 treatments is required to remove most visible hair. No common treatment protocol exists and it depends on the equipment used and patient skin type. The area to be treated should be clean shaven and free of sunburn. Treatment sessions are usually 4 to 6 weeks apart. Treatments are often given in office by trained Clinicians.

Contrary to what is often claimed, photoepilation is not a permanent hair removal method but a permanent hair reduction method. Although IPL treatments will permanently reduce the total number of body hairs, they will not result in a permanent removal of all hair. This distinction is only relevant in the USA because of FDA wording.

Certain skin conditions, health irregularities, and medications can impact whether it is safe for a person to receive a light based hair removal treatment. Photosensitizing medications or damage to the skin are contraindications to treatment. Manufacturers of IPL devices, and laser should only be used on light to medium skin tones, and work best on darker hair.

The first use of a specific IPL system developed for hair removal is reported in the literature in 1997. Hair count reduction was found to be ~60% (12 weeks), 75% (1 year), and 60% (2 year). Various treatment protocols have been studied.

It is important to note that these studies utilized a variety of IPL devices on various skin areas, and used patients with varying hair and skin types. Thus the results are not directly comparable. In evaluating these results it is also important to remember that even a reduction of 75% indicates that 25% of the hair regrew after treatment. Permanent hair removal in these studies, as defined by the FDA, means the "long-term, stable reduction in the number of hairs re-growing after a treatment regime". The number of hairs re-growing must be stable over time greater than the duration of the complete growth cycle of hair follicles, which varies from four to twelve months by body location. No treatment to date has shown the ability to permanently eliminate all hair growth, however many patients experience satisfaction with a significant and permanent reduction.

A 2006 article in the journal "Lasers in Medical Science" compared IPL and both alexandrite and diode lasers. The review found no statistical difference in effectiveness, but a higher incidence of side effects with diode laser treatment. Hair reduction after 6 months was reported as 68.75% for alexandrite lasers, 71.71% for diode lasers, and 66.96% for IPL. Side effects were reported as 9.5% for alexandrite lasers, 28.9% for diode lasers, and 15.3% for IPL. All side effects were found to be temporary and even pigmentation changes returned to normal within 6 months.

IPL was first developed for vascular conditions. It is at least as effective as pulsed dye lasers and can penetrate deeper with reduced risk of purpura and hyperpigmentation. IPL can treat pigmented lesions with rapid recovery. Dyschromia can be cleared after repeated sessions. This is accomplished with photo aging treatment. A series of

IPL treatment can be used for facial rejuvenation, improving skin laxity and collagen production. IPL combined with facial injections can be used for dynamic rhytides. Home devices are available, but will never give the result of professional care and treatment.

IPL is employed in the treatment of a range of dermatological conditions including photo damage induced depigmentation and vascular changes, Poikiloderma of Civatte, rosacea, acne vulgaris, sebaceous gland hyperplasia, broken capillaries/telangiectasia, vascular lesions (small blood vessels), pigmented lesions (freckles, liver spots, birthmarks), melasma, actinic keratosis, photo rejuvenation, basal cell carcinoma, and Bowen's disease (squamous cell carcinoma).

CHAPTER 5

What are Lasers?

Laser stands for Light Amplification by Stimulated Emission of Radiation. There are many different types of lasers and each uses a different type of laser medium that is excited by some form of energy to produce visible light or invisible ultraviolet or infrared radiation.

WHAT ARE LASERS USED FOR?

Lasers can be used for a variety of purposes. Many times you don't even realize it but common items such as pointers, CD and DVD players have lasers and most barcode scanners will use a laser. For are purpose lasers have been used for surgical and non-surgical treatments. Lasers are used for the removal of hair, wrinkles, fine lines, tattoos, and certain birthmarks like Port Wine stain, fine spider-like veins along with reddish or brownish blotches that can occur on the skin in most cases from sun damage.

CAN LASERS BE HAZARDOUS?

The short answer is "yes," however, if used correctly, they can be quite safe and every effective. Laser light can be hazardous due to two characteristics.

A laser beam when emitted is very tight and does not grow in size as the beam travels in distance. What this means is the same degree of hazard can occur whether you are close by or far away.

The human eye can focus a laser beam to a very small and intense spot on the retina which can result in damage to your eye if precautions are not followed.

CAN LASER RADIATION CAUSE CANCER?

While some lasers emit radiation that is invisible to the eye such as ultraviolet or infrared radiation, many lasers emit radiation in the form of light. In general laser radiation is not in itself harmful and will behave much like ordinary light in its interaction with the body. You should not confuse laser radiation with ionizing x-rays or radiation from radioactive substances.

CAN ALL LASERS BE USED ON PATIENTS?

The answer is no. Some lasers are only for industrial or entertainment reasons. The FDA requires labels on most laser products that contain a warning about laser radiation along with other hazards. Most consumer lasers products are generally labeled class I, IIa, IIIa while professional use will have the laser labeled as class IIIb or class IV. For the most part the higher the category the more powerful the laser.

Currently the FDA allows several manufacturers to label their products for permanent hair reduction, but not permanent removal. What this really means is are bodies have different types of hair from coarse to very fine almost baby like hair and no system completely removes all hair permanently.

CHAPTER 6

What are neuromodulators?

BOTOX® Cosmetic is a prescription medicine that is injected into muscles and used to temporarily improve the look of moderate to severe forehead lines, crow's feet lines, and frown lines between the eyebrows in adults.

There has not been a confirmed serious case of spread of toxin effect when BOTOX® Cosmetic has been used at the recommended dose to treat frown lines, crow's feet lines, and/or forehead lines.

You should not receive Botox if you are allergic to any of the ingredients in BOTOX® Cosmetic had an allergic reaction to any other botulinum toxin product such as Myobloc® (rimabotulinumtoxinB), Dysport® (abobotulinumtoxinA), or Xeomin® (incobotulinumtoxinA); have a skin infection at the planned injection site.

Please inform your clinician if you have ALS or Lou Gehrig's disease, myasthenia gravis, or Lambert-Eaton syndrome, as you may be at increased risk of serious side effects including difficulty swallowing and difficulty breathing from typical doses of BOTOX® Cosmetic.

Please inform your clinician if you have plans to have surgery; had surgery on your face; have trouble raising your eyebrows; drooping eyelids; any other abnormal facial change; are pregnant or plan to become pregnant (it is not known if BOTOX® Cosmetic can harm your unborn baby); are breastfeeding or plan to (it is not known if BOTOX® Cosmetic passes into breast milk).

Please inform your clinician of any over the counter medication, prescriptions and or herbal supplement before any neuromodulator injection. Using BOTOX® Cosmetic with certain other medicines may cause serious side effects. Do not start any new medicines until you have told your clinician that you have received BOTOX® Cosmetic in the past.

Tell your clinician if you have received any other botulinum toxin product in the last 4 months; have received injections of botulinum toxin such as Myobloc®, Dysport®, or Xeomin® in the past (tell your Clinician exactly which product you received); have recently received an antibiotic by injection; take muscle relaxants; take an allergy or cold medicine; take a sleep medicine; take aspirin-like products or blood thinners.

Side effects of BOTOX® Cosmetic include: dry mouth; discomfort or pain at the injection site; tiredness; headache; neck pain; and eye problems: double vision, blurred vision, decreased eyesight, drooping eyelids and eyebrows, swelling of your eyelids and dry eyes.

You may begin noticing results within 24 to 48 hours for moderate to severe frown lines starting to disappear, with results lasting up to 4 months.

Your clinician may use ice to numb the treatment area. If you are concerned about discomfort, your clinician may apply a topical numbing cream before administering your treatment. If a numbing cream is requested we suggest your arrive at your appointment at least 30 minutes ahead of your scheduled appointment. A clinician will discuss your treatment goals and perform a facial analysis to determine appropriate treatment areas for you to consider.

BOTOX® Cosmetic is a technique-sensitive treatment. You should not lose the ability to show expression when you are treated by someone who is licensed and trained.

Treatment requires minimal downtime or recovery; it's often called a *lunchtime procedure*. You'll be able to go about your normal routine immediately after you have completed your treatment.

Your cost not only includes the price of the product, but more importantly, the skill and expertise of the clinical professional who is administering your treatment.

BOTOX® Cosmetic is a technique-sensitive treatment—look for someone who is licensed and trained and has experience treating patients with BOTOX® Cosmetic.

CHAPTER 7

What are Fillers?

In most cases fillers are composed of Hyaluronic acid (HA). This is a naturally occurring substance that delivers nutrients to the skin, helping the skin retain moisture and softness and adding volume. Fillers add volume to different areas of the face to lift cheeks, smooth parentheses lines, plump up the lip along with many other options being available. The results should be subtle and can be long lasting depending on the type of product used.

Over time your face will change in many ways and is part of the normal aging process. You should remember genetics and environmental factors also play a role in how your face and skin will age. In most cases you may start to notice changes in your skin such as wrinkles with the medical term rhytides. In many cases what you may be noticing is age related mid-face volume loss. What this means is gravity is setting in and things are starting to fall! Your cheeks look flatter and skin appears to be sagging. What is really happening is over time your skin loses some of their building blocks (like collagen and HA). This naturally occurring loss of products in skin structure happens throughout the entire body, even including the lips.

You should ask your healthcare clinician to do a facial analysis so we fully understand your concerns to make sure a non-surgical option is right for you.

Our job to help you understand that there are many products on the market and each product can be used in many different areas of the body but in most cases each product is best suited for a particular area and each product will last a particular period of time. The take home is no product last forever so continuous maintenance provides the best long lasting results.

In most cases certain filler products will be ideal for fine lines, while other products will be better for deeper lines and wrinkles. Some products are ideal for the cheek area, while some products are ideal for the nasolabial fold area and some products are ideal for the lips. building blocks (like collagen and HA). This naturally occurring loss of products in skin structure happens throughout the entire body, even including the lips.

We recommend you don't just look at price but the artistic ability of your clinician and experience.

Consider the following, product A last 24 months and is $1200.00 and product B is $600.00 but last 4 months in actuality even though product B is less expensive than product A, product A is a better value long term. The art is having your clinician along with your input select the correct product for the correct location to provide the best long term results.

In most cases, the procedure is mostly pain free; however, the client will receive an injection. Most fillers have had an anesthetic similar to a dental injection as part of the filler so the area will get and be numb making the procedure quite comfortable.

In most cases it will take 2-4 days for the product to settle in, and the results generally improve over the first week.

The following are some important information tips to help you decide if fillers are the right decision for you.

Do not use these products if you have a history of multiple severe allergies or severe allergic reactions (anaphylaxis), or if you are allergic to lidocaine or the Gram-positive bacterial proteins used in these products.

- Tell your Clinician if you are pregnant or breastfeeding. The safety of these products for use during pregnancy or while breastfeeding has not been studied

- Tell your clinician if you have a history of excessive scarring (e.g., hypertrophic scarring and keloid formations) or pigmentation disorders, as use of these products may result in additional scars or changes in pigmentation

- Tell your clinician if you are planning other laser treatments or a chemical peel, as there is a possible risk of inflammation at the treatment site if these procedures are performed after treatment

- Patients who experience skin injury near the site of injection with this product may be at a higher risk for side effects

- Tell your Clinician if you are on immunosuppressive therapy used to decrease the body's immune response, as use of these products may result in an increased risk of infection

- Tell your Clinician if you are using medications that can prolong bleeding, such as aspirin, ibuprofen, or other blood thinners, as this may result in increased bruising or bleeding at the injection site

- Minimize strenuous exercise, exposure to extensive sun or heat, and alcoholic beverages within the first 24 hours following treatment.

- The most commonly reported side effects with injectable gels included injection site redness, swelling, pain, tenderness, firmness, lumps/bumps, bruising, discoloration, and itching. Some dryness to the skin area has been reported. Most side effects will be moderate and last 2 to 4 weeks.

- One of the risks of using these products is unintentional injection into a blood vessel, and while rare, the complications can be serious and may be permanent. These complications, which have been reported for facial injections, can include vision abnormalities, blindness, stroke, temporary scabs, or permanent scarring.

- As with all skin injection procedures, there is a risk of infection.

CHAPTER 8

HydraFacial

HydraFacial is a facial on steroids! It is considered an advanced medical grade skin care treatment that can be used anywhere on the body, but in most cases will be done on your face and back. It will focus on improving fine lines and wrinkles along with treating congested, oily and acne prone skin, along with skin that is suffering from rosacea, hyperpigmentation. The HydraFacial will soften the appearance of large pores along with improving your skin's texture, tone and tightness while repairing sun damaged areas.

HydraFacial is a hydra dermabrasion facial combing cleansing, exfoliation, extraction, hydration and antioxidant protection in a non-invasive process in 30-60 minutes to make your skin clearer and more beautiful.

HOW IT WORKS:

CLEANSE + PEEL

Uncover a new layer of skin with gentle exfoliation and relaxing resurfacing.

EXTRACT + HYDRATE

Remove debris from pores with painless suction. Nourish with intense moisturizers that quench skin.

FUSE + PROTECT

HydraFacial is an invigorating treatment that can be given in as little as 30 minutes. It delivers long-term skin health and can be tailored to meet the specific needs of all skin types. It offers instant, noticeable results with no downtime or irritation. The HydraFacial treatment removes dead skin cells and extracts impurities while simultaneously bathing the new skin with cleansing, hydrating and moisturizing serums. The treatment is soothing, refreshing, non-irritating and immediately effective.

Hydration is the foundation of healthy, radiant skin. Irritation of the skin has been proven to increase signs of aging. HydraFacial is a hydrating and non-irritating treatment. The HydraFacial treatment is designed for all skin types. Even the most sensitive skin easily tolerates the HydraFacial treatment. Your Clinician or skincare professional may choose specific treatment serums and/or customize the treatment for your unique skin conditions and needs. Consult your skincare professional for a skin evaluation and sensitivity test

Our goal is to help support you in a balanced lifestyle. That's why HydraFacial is a fast, efficient treatment that takes as little as 30 minutes. You may put on makeup and return to your normal activities right after the treatment since there is no downtime.

Many clients report seeing visible skin refinement and an even, radiant skin tone after just one treatment. The smooth results and hydration may last 5 to 7 days or even longer. We don't believe in quick fixes, so one treatment per month is recommended for improving the appearance of fine lines, wrinkles, and brown spots, oily and congested skin. Continued HydraFacial treatments are highly recommended to maintain skin health results.

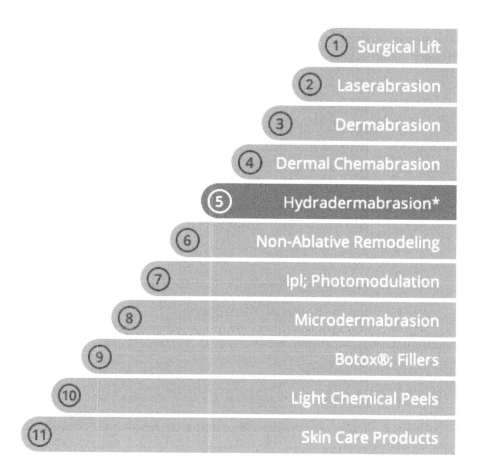

①	Surgical Lift
②	Laserabrasion
③	Dermabrasion
④	Dermal Chemabrasion
⑤	Hydradermabrasion*
⑥	Non-Ablative Remodeling
⑦	Ipl; Photomodulation
⑧	Microdermabrasion
⑨	Botox®; Fillers
⑩	Light Chemical Peels
⑪	Skin Care Products

The ergonomically designed, dual-functioning hand piece gives you control over serum type and flow, enabling the clinican to tailor the treatment to different skin types and concerns. In addition, each treatment uses a series of unique tips – each with multiple edges to gently exfoliate the skin several times each pass, achieving better, more even results.

The unique spiral design of the Hydro Peel® Tips used in conjunction with the HydraFacial MD® proprietary vacuum technology and serums creates a vortex effect to easily dislodge and remove impurities while simultaneously introducing hydrating skin solutions with potent antioxidants. This multi-step process includes

Vortex-Exfoliation™, Vortex-Peel™, Vortex-Extraction™, Vortex-Boost™, and Vortex-Fusion.

Antioxidants… we can't get enough of them! Antioxidants are persistent in fighting against free radical damage while nourishing skin as they boost hydration and enhance skin tone evenness. Phytonutrient-rich products feature a powerhouse combination of antioxidants that work to restore beautifully healthy skin.

TREATMENT & TAKE-HOME WITH ANTIOXIDANTS INCLUDE:

Activ™ Foaming Cleanser

Antiox +™/ Antiox +™ with Even Tone & Firming

Award-Winning Antiox-6™ / Antiox-6™ Daily

Britenol® / Britenol® Intensive Spot Corrector

Pur Moist™ Oil-Free

UV Smart® Daily SPF 40

Growth factors are natural proteins that assist in a variety of activities in the body especially in the skin's healing process. Young skin stay smooth and resilient longer because growth factors keep the skin nourished. However as we age growth factors decrease and create signs of aging skin. When having a HydraFacial the product CTGF will be incorporated into your skin to provide healthy glowing appearance while reducing the signs of aging.

Growth Factors, really? Growth Factors are natural proteins, commonly known as "Peptides" and a choice ingredient in minimizing the appearance of aging skin. With HydraFacial MD® treatments and take-home products containing a multi-peptide blend, skin will be rejuvenated. These powerful amino acids work hard to reduce the appearance of fine lines and wrinkles, leaving skin looking younger and feeling refreshed.

TREATMENT & TAKE-HOME WITH PEPTIDES INCLUDE:

Antiox +™/ Antiox +™ with Even Tone & Firming

DermaBuilder™ / DermaBuilder™ Daily

ETX™ Age-Refining Eye Cream heals the skin. However, factor levels decrease, and will capture naturally derived growth factors and sealed Brightening Agents: it's inevitable. As we age, dark spots and discoloration become more noticeable and skin becomes uneven in tone due to a variety of factors. It's time to awaken dull skin with Britenol®. This specially formulated spot corrector treatment and take-home product will leave skin radiant with a more even complexion.

Treatment & Take-Home with Brightening Agents Include:

Antiox +™/ Antiox +™ with Even Tone & Firming

Britenol® / Britenol® Intensive Spot Corrector

NEW FORMULA, CTACIDS

While some may find the very words acid peel a bit daunting, we believe they provide excellent benefits. Glycolic, Salicylic, and Lactic acids are used frequently in HydraFacial MD® treatments and take-home products. The primary function of these acids include gently exfoliating skin by sloughing away dead skin cells. HydraFacial MD® acid peel formulations are great for all skin types, especially those with oily and congested skin.

Treatment & Take-Home with Acids Include:

Activ-4™

Beta-HD™ / Beta-HD™ Daily

GlySal™

CHAPTER 9

Hair Removal

Hair removal, also known as epilation or depilation, is the deliberate removal of body hair. Hair typically grows all over the human body. Hair can become more visible during and after puberty, and men tend to have thicker, more visible body hair than women. Both men and women have visible hair on the head, eyebrows, eyelashes, armpits, pubic region, arms, and legs; men and some women also have thicker hair on their face, abdomen, back and chest. Hair does not generally grow on the lips, the underside of the hands or feet or on certain areas of the genitalia.

Hair removal can be accomplished by many methods and all methods have some advantages and disadvantages. Let our clinicians guide you through the options and techniques that are available and help you choose the options that are best for your individual needs.

Trichology is the study of hair and its diseases. Hair is affected by age and hormones. Hair formation begins before birth. The hair on a fetus is called lanugo and after birth is replaced by either vellus or terminal hairs which are stronger and pigmented. Vellus hair is very fine and soft and is what is usually seen and grows on a woman's cheek sometimes referred to as peach fuzz. It is not recommended to remove these types of hair as doing so can allow the follicles to start producing new terminal type hair which is both coarse and darker. It is, therefore, not recommended to tweeze, shave or wax these fine hairs.

Hair comes from a protein called keratin which is produced from the hair follicle, and the hair follicle is a mass of epidermal cells forming a small tube or canal which extends into the dermis. A strand of hair is divided into two parts, the root and the shaft. The root anchors the hair to skin cells and is part of the hair located at the bottom of the follicle below the surface of the skin. The shaft is defined as the part of the hair located above the surface of the skin.

Hair growth occurs in three stages. The Anagen phase or growth stage in which new hair is produced. The Catagen phase is the transition stage of hair growth. The last stage is called the Telogen phase or final stage of hair growth or resting stage, and it is in this stage that the hair starts to fall out.

Several appointments will be necessary for hair removal/reduction as the body is producing hair in each of the three cycles, while hair reduction can only occur during the Anagen stage.

Methods of hair removal fall into two broad categories, temporary or permanent. Permanent hair removal occurs when the papilla is destroyed which inhibits re-growth. Any technique that can destroy papilla will result in permanent hair loss.

Hair removal options include electrolysis which is comprised of three methods Galvanic, Thermolysis and Blend. The Galvanic method uses direct current which will cause chemical decomposition of the hair follicle. A needle is inserted into the hair follicle, an electrical charge is applied which transforms the saline moisture inside the follicle into sodium hydroxide (or lye) along with hydrogen and chlorine gas. These chemicals destabilize the follicle wall through a chemical reaction and allow the hair to be removed. This technique relies on the moisture in the skin to be effective and is generally a much slower technique than Thermolysis.

Thermolysis is a method that uses high frequency current to produce heat which coagulates and destroys the hair follicle through a process is called electrocoagulation. An alternating current passes through a needle causing the water molecules to vibrate producing heat which destroys the papilla.

The Blend technique is a combination of both methods; direct and alternating current is used to destroy the hair follicle resulting in hair loss. The Blend method tends to be quicker than the Galvanic or Thermolysis options.

In addition to electrolysis, other treatments intended to destroy the hair follicle include Laser and Pulsed Light options. These techniques tend to be faster and less uncomfortable and have been used in some shape or form since 1980's. Many different laser can achieve hair reduction such as the Diode laser, Alexandrite laser and Nd: Yag laser. All lasers are attracted to pigments called chromophores, so the darker the hair the better the results, and the lighter the hair the poorer the results. What this means in darker skinned individuals is that there is an increased chance for PIH or post inflammatory hyperpigmentation due to the lack of contrast between the color of the skin and color of the hair.

Intense Pulsed Light is slightly different from traditional laser which are a solid beam of light however the IPL produces a quick flash of light and these short powerful burst of energy shatter the hair follicle without allowing heat to build up and burn the surrounding skin.

The temporary methods of hair removal are either Depilation or epilation. Depilation is a process of removing hair at or near the level of the skin and examples would be shaving and chemical products. Epilation is the process of removing hair from the bottom of the follicle by breaking contact between the hair bulb and the papilla so the hair is pulled out of the follicle. Example of epilation would be tweezing, waxing, depilatories and sugaring.

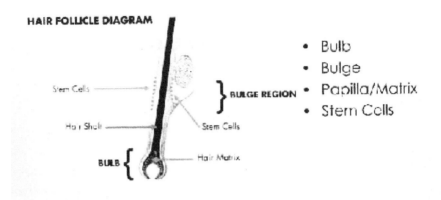

HAIR FOLLICLE DIAGRAM

- Bulb
- Bulge
- Papilla/Matrix
- Stem Cells

Stem Cells

Hair Shaft

BULGE REGION

Stem Cells

BULB

Hair Matrix

Region	Phases of Cycle (%)		Phase Duration, Weeks		Average Length of Developed Anagen Hair Follicle
	Anagen	Telogen	Anagen	Telogen	mm
Lip	65	35	8-19	6-7	1.8
Chin	70	30	48-50	10-12	3
Cheek	50-70	30-50	N/A	N/A	3
Bikini	30-40	54-70	16-18	12-14	4
Axillae	30-40	54-70	16	12	4
Arm	20-30	69-80	3-13	11-18	3
Leg	20-40	54-80	16-22	11-24	3.2

When deciding on Hair removal with any technique it is important to understand Cautionary and Exclusionary issues in your past and present medical history. The following is list of each that your clinician will review with you when considering IPL and or Laser hair removal.

CAUTIONARY ISSUES

1. A history of herpes infection that is active

2. The use of exfoliates such as Retinoid within the last two weeks

3. Uncontrolled hormonal changes

4. Changes in medical history

EXCLUSIONARY ISSUES

1. A history of seizures

2. Pregnancy

3. Undiagnosed lesions

4. Waxing, tweezing, epilation within the last 4-6 weeks

5. Immunosuppression medication or medical condition

6. Active infection

7. Blood thinners or coagulation issues

8. Open Lesions in the area of treatment

9. Active tan within 4-6 weeks of treatment

After your clinician reviews cautionary and exclusionary conditions we will review in more detail your current and past medical history, along with review and have you sign an informed consent. We strongly recommend the daily use of a broad spectrum sunscreen with a SPF of at least 45, since your skin can become hypersensitive to UVA and UVB radiation from the sun after IPL or Laser treatments.

You and your clinician should be looking for clinical end points to determine the effectiveness of your treatment. Some of these clinical endpoints are the following.

1. Mild to moderate perifollicular edema

2. Mild to moderate erythema or redness

3. Darkening of freckles

HOME CARE INSTRUCTIONS AFTER YOUR TREATMENT ARE THE FOLLOWING:

1. Apply cold gel packs as needed to provide comfort and reduce irritation for about 15 minutes every hour until symptoms have calmed down.

2. You can expect a mild sunburn like sensation in the area of treatment and this can last anywhere from 2-72 hours.

3. You can expect prolonged redness, crusting or blistering which could occur but fairly rare. We have you consider an antibiotic ointment or moisturizing lotion to be applied twice a day to the treated area.

4. In some instances your clinician may recommend steroidal creams after treatment.

Remember all treatments will make your skin more susceptible to sunlight and precaution must be strictly followed. Consider the following information to help you avoid complication and post treatment issues.

1. The average person receives around 18 hours of unexpected sun exposure a week

2. You should of avoided sun exposure to the treatment area for at least 4 weeks prior to treatment

3. Sun exposure during the treatment course may decrease the efficacy of the treatment and increase unwanted side effects

4. Sun avoidance and the use of a SPF 45 sunscreen or higher throughout your treatment is highly recommended. This increases the chances that no skin color changes will occur.

5. Apply a moisturizer to dry and or itchy skin twice a day until symptoms resolve.

6. You can expect the appearance of hair growth or stubble within 7-30 days after treatment but this is not new growth.

Because of the different hair growth stages additional treatment sessions will be necessary.

7. Clipping or shaving of the treatment area is permitted.

8. You should avoid excessive exercise, pools, Jacuzzis, saunas and hot tubs for 7 days or until redness has resolved.

9. Avoid picking or removing scabs or crusted areas to reduce or avoid scarring.

CHAPTER 10

Wrinkle Sun Damage
Red and Brown Spot Removal
Scar and Small Vein Reduction

During this chapter many subjects will be addressed. Let's start by talking about Non-Ablative Fractional Laser treatment for skin resurfacing. The goal is to provide controlled damage to your skin so the reparative process will take place stimulating new collagen and make your skin young and healthier looking.

THE FOLLOWING WILL BE SOME APPLICATIONS FOR YOUR CONSIDERATIONS.

1. Skin resurfacing

2. Soft tissue coagulation

3. Acne Scar and Surgical Scar reduction and or removal

4. Melasma or darkening pigmentation sometimes associated with hormonal changes

5. Striae or stretch marks

Stratum corneum remains intact which allows for rapid healing.

Healing occurs from viable untreated tissue between the columns of coagulated zones.

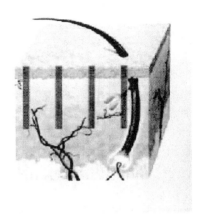

YOU AND YOUR CLINICIAN WILL NEED TO FORMULATE A TREATMENT PLAN AND OR STRATEGY WHICH WILL TAKE IN THE FOLLOWING CONSIDERATIONS.

1. Consideration of the amount of correction needed and the relative thickness of your skin.

2. The amount of pressure or compression that will be used when applying the laser tip or IPL tip to the treatment area.

3. The setting necessary to get optimum results which will include energy level, pulse duration and type of laser or IPL to be used.

4. Past and present medical history must be reviewed.

5. Determination of whether topical anesthesia will be used or not in the treatment area.

6. How much treatment will be necessary and during each treatment how many passes will be necessary on the treatment area. In most cases no more than two passes will be done to avoid overheating the tissue in the area being treated.

7. In general lower energy means lower coverage so expect 3-4 treatments with each treatment 1-4 weeks apart. For higher energy and higher coverage consider 1-2 treatments and 4-6 weeks between treatments.

46

DESIRABLE CLINICAL ENDPOINTS TO BE EXPECTED ARE.

1. Transient erythema and or edema immediately post treatment. (redness and swelling)

2. Bronzing (brown debris) may develop a few day post treatment.

POSSIBLE SIDE EFFECTS:

1. A low risk of prolonged itching, redness and blistering.

2. Acne breakouts

3. A risk of hyperpigmentation, hypopigmentation, burns, bruising or blistering may occur in which some scarring could occur.

4. A risk of infection

5. Please advise your clinician of any post treatment side effects.

POST TREATMENT GUIDELINES:

1. Avoid unprotected sun exposure

2. Avoid excessive exercise for 1-3 days after treatment

3. Consider cool packs immediately post treatment 15 minutes every hour as needed.

4. Avoid makeup and moisturizer for at least 24 hours to avoid acne breakouts.

5. Consider gentle cleansing with non-irritating cosmetics

6. No retinoid 2 weeks prior and throughout the course of treatment.

7. After 24 hours you can consider a thin layer of occlusive ointment during the healing process to help minimize TWL or transepidermal water loss.

8. Consider 10 minute soaks to gently remove bronzing debris

9. The treated area should not be picked at or scrubbed to avoid scarring.

Your clinician will review Cautionary and Exclusionary criteria before treatment is considered and the following are some area you should be aware of.

CAUTIONARY CRITERIA:

1. History of Herpes I or II within the treatment area.

2. History of heat urticaria

3. Diabetes

4. Cosmetic dermal fillers, neuromodulators (Botox) and or implants in the area of treatment. You should avoid these products 2-4 weeks prior to and after treatment.

5. A history of vitiligo, eczema, psoriasis, allergic dermatitis, autoimmune diseases, on immunocompromised medication or condition, any diseases that affect collagen including Ehlers-Danios syndrome and scleroderma or any condition that may affect you and your response to treatment.

6. Tretinoin, Retin-A, Renova and exfoliating products should be discontinued at least 2 weeks before and throughout the course of treatments. The use of Isotretinoin (Accutane) within the last 6-12 months, The use of systemic steroids and anticoagulants at least two weeks prior to treatment.

7. Undiagnosed pigmented lesions

8. Medication both prescription and non-prescriptions including herbal and natural remedies that may have photosensitivity associated with them.

EXCLUSIONARY CRITERIA:

9. A history of light induced seizures

10. Pregnancy

11. Skin cancer

12. Active infection

13. Open lesions or sores in the treatment area

14. Blood disorders

15. A history of keloid formation

Your treatment will take between 15-60 minutes depending on the size of the area to be treated and in most cases only mild or moderate discomfort can be expected during the treatment. In most cases no topical anesthetic will be necessary however if you are concerned topical anesthetic can be applied about 20-30 minutes prior to treatment.

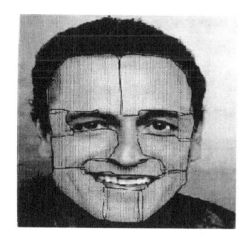

Treatment Zones

Deliver all passes to a limited area before moving to the next.

This will allow all energy to be delivered before significant edema occurs.

49

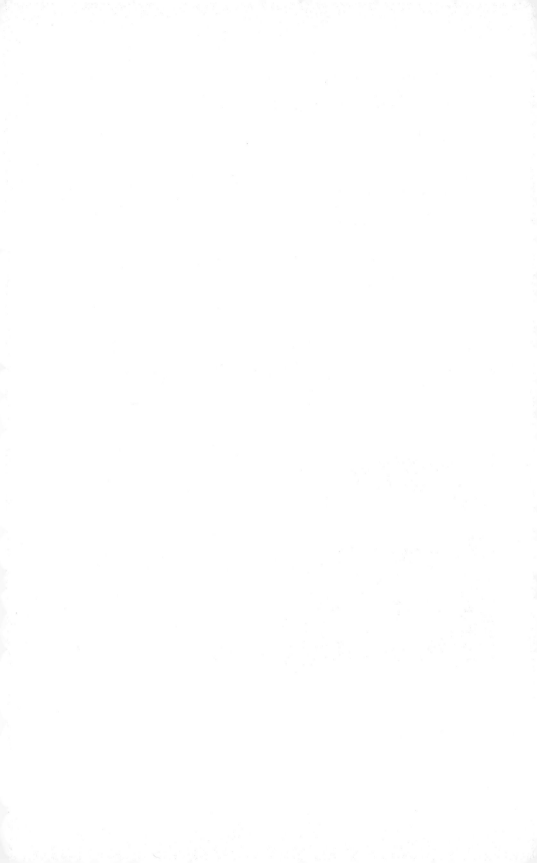

CHAPTER 11

Tattoo removal

If you are considering tattoo removal, here are some interesting facts. It is estimated that about 85% of people over the age of 45 are seeking tattoo removal. The biggest reason is that they have started to fade and no longer look as good as they once did. Another reason is that your personal life has changed and you no longer LOVE John or Mary!

Most tattoos are made of many different colors; the most common colors being black, blue, red, green, orange and yellow. When considering tattoo removal you must seek a system and procedure that will allow all colors to be addressed. If the laser system does not work for a variety of wavelengths, you will see some improvement; but, in many cases results may be disappointing.

There are many types of tattoo inks. These inks are not regulated, which makes it very difficult to formulate exact protocols for this type of procedure. In addition, the depth of the tattoo may differ by each tattoo artist. Every tattoo will require an evaluation, and may take several visits or treatments to produce the desired result.

In most cases, a laser will be used to remove a tattoo. Since all lasers are attracted to pigment, the laser may not always distinguish between tattoo pigment and skin pigment. One of the first steps to be determined by your clinician is to evaluate your skin type. There are six types of skin that are universally accepted when being evaluated for laser treatment. Skin types are determined by using the Fitzpatrick Skin Scale and are listed as follows:

Skin type I - Light color hair and eyes, always burns and never tans

Skin type II - Light skin and light colored hair, usually burns but can tan with difficulty

Skin type III - Darker eyes and slight coloring to the skin and sometimes burns but usually will tan

Skin type IV - Dark eye color and definitive darkening of the skin and rarely burns and tans easily

Skin type V - Dark hair and eye color and very rarely burns

Skin type VI - Very dark hair and eyes along with very dark skin color

There are several different lasers that are available for tattoo removal. Many of the topics were discussed in chapter 5 however when it comes to tattoo removal you may have heard the terms: Nano and Pico. These terms refer to the amount of time a laser fires or expresses its energy. In order to remove a tattoo, the clinician will need to break down the ink, but attempt to avoid damaging the skin.

Nano generally means that the laser is firing at one billionth of a second, and Pico means that the laser is firing at one trillionth of a second. The concept is that at one trillionth of a second, the laser system is not really using HEAT to destroy the tattoo, but POWER. It is actually taking the tiny granules of ink in the tattoo and pulverizing them into incredibly small particles so that the body will excrete these pigmented particles out of the body through the lymphatic system. Using a laser system that operates using power will treat the tattoo faster, and with much less risk of damaging the skin.

PRETREATMENT CONSIDERATIONS BETWEEN YOU AND YOUR CLINICIAN ARE THE FOLLOWING:

1. Is the tattoo old or new? For example, if the tattoo is dull with indistinct and blurred margins it is most likely an old tattoo, and if it has sharp and distinct lines with bright colors, it is more likely a new tattoo.

2. Is your tattoo deep or superficial? In most cases if your tattoo artist placed the tattoo deeper into your skin it may take longer or more treatments to remove

3. If your tattoo is new it is suggested you wait at least 3 months before considering to remove it. We have all done things we regret the next day, and the placement of a tattoo sometimes falls into that category!

4. The laser will impact tattoo ink by fragmentation or breaking the ink into small particles

5. Some of the tattoo ink may be stored in the regional lymph nodes and some ink will be cleared and excreted through the lymphatic system or through transdermal transport.

6. When considering tattoo removal, remember it will be accomplished through gradual fading. The speed and success of this fading will depend on many factors including tattoo size, depth, density of pigment, location, along with your age and skin condition.

7. Cosmetic inks used for enhancing eyebrows or other areas may oxidize, darken, or change color from laser exposure.

8. Multiple wavelengths may be necessary to address the different colors of your tattoo.

9. In most cases we suggest doing a test spot in an inconspicuous area to evaluate how your skin will react

The following are some pre-treatment guidelines that will be suggested.

1. When having your tattoo treated please follow all instructions

2. Please shave the night before or morning of treatment if the area is hair bearing

3. No sun exposure for 4 weeks prior to or after the tattoo procedure

4. If you have a cosmetic tattoo and it is present in the area of the tattoo we want to remove we will generally stay at least two fingerbreadths away from that area to avoid potential darkening of that area.

5. The area of treatment will be cleaned with 70% isopropyl alcohol and then allowed to dry

6. In most cases we will need to do a test spot and evaluate that test spot 4-6 weeks later to see how the tattoo reacted along with your skin.

7. When a laser is used to remove a tattoo in many cases the energy in the laser can create a plume or fumes, and we may use a vacuum system to evacuate these potentially harmful by products from your treatment

Post treatment suggestions are as follows:

1. Use cold gel packs until heat dissipates

2. Keep area moist with a thin layer of ointment such as Aquaphor or your clinicians choice of ointment

3. Wash the treated area gently with soap and water

4. Do not soak area treated

5. Do not shave the treated area if crusting is evident

6. Avoid contact sports or any other activity that could cause injury to the treated area

POSSIBLE SIDE EFFECTS:

1. Discomfort, redness, swelling, pinpoint bleeding, blistering, scabbing, crusting and bruising

2. In some cases you may see pustules, skin burns, hypopigmentation, hyperpigmentation, scarring, infection and or an allergic reaction the breakdown of the ink. Pigmentation changes usually resolve within 1-12 months. Blisters are not caused by heat but by mechanically induced pressure waves that break up tattoo pigment granules. Do not pop blisters or tear skin away but allow to heal on their own.

3. In most cases these are transient side effects that will resolve without any intervention or time.

CAUTIONARY CRITERIA ARE AS FOLLOWS FOR LASER AND LIGHT BASED TREATMENT OF TATTOO REMOVAL:

1. Certain types of medication such as blood thinners, systemic steroids, topical retinoid and Tretinoin

2. Blood disorders

3. Poor healing capabilities

4. Having treatment for skin cancer, active infection or immunocompromised, a history of radiation therapy in the area to be treated, active bacterial or viral infection or any inflammatory condition in the area to be treated.

5. A history of skin photosensitivity or history of hypertrophic scars or keloid formation

6. Heat urticaria

7. An unwillingness or unable to follow post treatment instructions.

8. The use of fillers and or neuromodulators (Botox) 2-4 weeks prior to treatment or during treatment in the area to be treated.

9. Diabetes

10. Menstrual dysfunction polycystic ovarian syndrome or PCOS

11. The use of tanning beds or spray tans in the area to be treated 2-4 weeks prior to or during your treatment.

12. In some cases paradoxical hair growth has been noted

EXCLUSIONARY CRITERIA FOR TATTOO REMOVAL:

1. Hypersensitivity to light in the near infrared wavelength region

2. Taking medication or products that are known to increase sensitivity to sunlight

3. Seizure disorder triggered by light

4. Have taken oral isotretinoin such as Accutane within the last 6 months.

5. If you have an active localized or systemic infection or open wound in the area to be treated

6. The presence of Nevi (birthmarks) that could have a predisposition to cancer

7. Active Herpes

8. Are receiving Gold therapy

9. Are pregnant or breastfeeding or (lactating)

EXPECTED CLINICAL ENDPOINT AFTER TATTOO REMOVAL TREATMENT IS AS FOLLOWS:

1. Slight epidermal whitening or frosting of the area

2. This frosting effect will not be as evident after multiple treatments

3. In some cases your tattoo will appear yellow, gray, beige or possibly even other shades

4. Expect perilesional erythema or redness and edema or swelling

5. If you see purpura or bruising or pinpoint bleeding during the treatment your clinician may just need to lower the power setting.

In most cases, your tattoo removal appointments will be short, usually only a few minutes based on the size of the tattoo being removed. In many cases, most clients will need several appointments to complete the treatment. Each visit will be between 4-8 weeks apart. In most cases the discomfort will be similar to a rubber band snap your skin. To imply no pain would be misleading, but with treatment times so short most clients will not require any topical anesthesia.

CHAPTER 12

Body Re-contouring

Currently there are four techniques for the removal of subcutaneous body fat or adipose tissue. Those options are Laser, RF (or radiofrequency), Cold (or hypothermic) treatment, and Surgery. These four options all have the same goal: destroy fat cells and reduce adipose tissue under the chin or the submental region, inner thighs, outer thighs, abdomen or stomach region, and love handles or flank area. Research indicates that we can expect between 24% and 37% reduction in subcutaneous fat in the above mentioned regions.

Ideally we look for a system that not only reduces fat cells, but can tighten the loosen skin after your procedures. Consider a system that reduces the chance of postoperative complications and discomfort, and one that will be completed in a timely fashion. In most cases treatment is completed in two – three sessions each session 25-30 minutes in duration and each session 4-6 weeks apart. Results will be seen over a 3 month period of time. During this time the fat cells or adipose tissue will be excreted or eliminated through your lymphatic system.

Even with diet and exercise stubborn fat seems impossible to lose. Light based body contouring technology targets and destroys fat in problem areas to help you achieve a slimmer appearance.

THE OBJECT TO TREATMENT IS THE FOLLOWING:

1. Permanent reduction in fat cells

2. Customizable treatments

3. Safety for all skin colors

4. Natural looking results by blending

5. FDA cleared treatment

You can expect your appointment to be between 25-60 minutes. After treatment you expect to resume your normal daily activities.

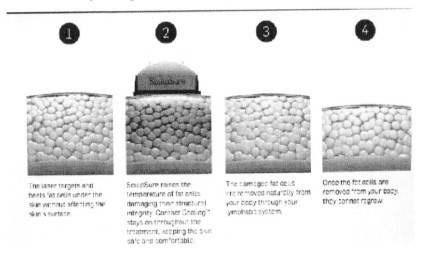

The following diagrams offer you some ideas of how and where we will place the laser sensors to re-contour your body shape!

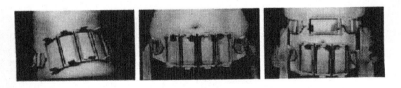

Your clinician will review your medical history, determine your problem areas, and calculate your Body Mass Index (BMI) to determine if you are a candidate for treatment. This calculation will be determined by your current height and weight.

Your clinician will then determine your specific body type to help determine the number of sensors and placement of sensors to determine the required amount of appointment time and cost of your treatment. For best results we strongly recommend treating to completion, which really means after determining area, and body type we know how many sensors will be needed and each area will require 25 minutes of treatment on average. At no point at time can any system currently on the market provide more than four sensors at one time. Depending on what you are trying to accomplish, additional visits will be necessary, or longer appointments will be necessary, to treat multiple areas. For example, in order to treat the lower abdomen and the upper abdomen in the same visit, each area will require one session, each approximately 25 minutes. In addition, each area may possibly require four sensors to the area. Commonly, fees are based upon the area treated, by the number of sensors required, or a combination of both.

BEFORE YOUR APPOINTMENT CONSIDER THE FOLLOWING STEPS AND RECOMMENDATIONS:

1. Your skin should be fee of creams or lotions

2. If you have thick hair in the area to be treated please shave or trim area before your appointment

3. Please wear plain black underwear and or bra to provide consistent pre and post- operative photos

4. Have a light meal and drink 2-3 glasses of water an hour before your treatment

5. At the beginning of treatment you will feel a cooling sensation which keeps your skin safe and comfortable

6. Two minutes into the treatment you will start to feel peaks of warmth followed by cooling

7. Four minutes into the treatment you will feel deep warmth and tingling. Some clients feel a sensation of pressure or squeezing and this is okay and expected. The warmth will build in order to reach the correct sensation of heat in order to kill your fat cells.

YOUR TREATMENT WILL FALL INTO FIVE ZONES WITH ZONE FOUR BEING THE GOAL TO KILL YOUR FAT CELL AND GET THE BEST RESULTS. THE ZONES ARE OFTEN DESCRIBED AS FOLLOWS:

1. Zone one- pleasant cool feeling

2. Zone two- gentle warming and cooling

3. Zone three- Tingly with short intervals of warm and cooling

4. Zone four- The zone where all the work is being done. In this zone you should experience prickling, pinching, pressure, and longer peaks of moderate deep heat and cooling. This is where you are getting your best results.

5. Zone five- Usually a zone which cannot be tolerated; we want to avoid Zone 5

WHEN YOUR TREATMENT IS COMPLETE YOU CAN CONSIDER THE FOLLOWING HOME CARE INSTRUCTIONS:

1. Gently massage the area twice a day for -10 minutes

2. Be sure to drink plenty of water every day

3. Exercise will help damaged fat cells move through the lymphatic system

4. Maintain healthy eating habits

5. You may experience mild redness, tenderness, swelling and tissue firmness which could last two weeks or longer.

PICTURED BELOW ARE THE THREE MAIN BODY TYPES FOR MALES AND FEMALES:

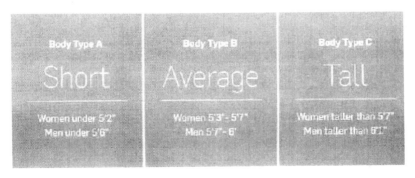

The following diagrams illustrate where the clinician will place the laser, how many attachments will be needed, and how long the procedure could take. Each body type: A, B, or C will have 1-3 specific types--labeled 1, 2, or 3.

BODY TYPE A ONE FEMALE

Body Type A1
Female
Height: 5'2"   Weight: 122 lbs

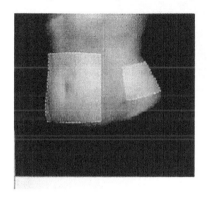

Treatment Plan

Series 1	Series 2
3 TREATMENT AREAS	3 TREATMENT AREAS
• Lower Abdomen	• Lower Abdomen
• Upper Abdomen	• Upper Abdomen
• Left & Right Flanks	• Left & Right Flanks
75 minutes	75 minutes

BODY TYPE A TWO FEMALE

Body Type A2
Female
Height: 4'11"   Weight: 138 lbs

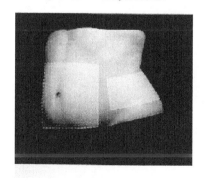

Treatment Plan

Series 1	Series 2
4 TREATMENT AREAS	4 TREATMENT AREAS
• Lower Abdomen	• Lower Abdomen
• Upper Abdomen	• Upper Abdomen
• Left Flank	• Left Flank
• Right Flank	• Right Flank
100 minutes	100 minutes

BODY TYPE A THREE FEMALE

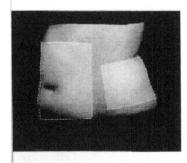

Body Type A3
Female
Height: 5'2"   Weight: 146 lbs

Treatment Plan

Series 1	Series 2	Series 3 (Subject to Patient)
6 TREATMENT AREAS	6 TREATMENT AREAS	6 TREATMENT AREAS
• Lower Abdomen	• Lower Abdomen	• Lower Abdomen
• Middle Abdomen	• Middle Abdomen	• Middle Abdomen
• Upper Abdomen	• Upper Abdomen	• Upper Abdomen
• Lower Left Flank	• Lower Left Flank	• Lower Left Flank
• Lower Right Flank	• Lower Right Flank	• Lower Right Flank
• Upper Left & Right Flanks	• Upper Left & Right Flanks	• Upper Left & Right Flanks
150 minutes	**150 minutes**	**150 minutes**

BODY TYPE B ONE FEMALE

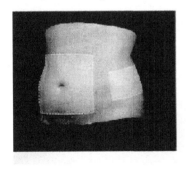

Body Type B1
Female
Height: 5'6"   Weight: 146 lbs

Treatment Plan

Series 1	Series 2
3 TREATMENT AREAS	3 TREATMENT AREAS
• Lower Abdomen	• Lower Abdomen
• Upper Abdomen	• Upper Abdomen
• Left & Right Flanks	• Left & Right Flanks
75 minutes	**75 minutes**

64

BODY TYPE B TWO FEMALE

Body Type B2
Female
Height: 5'5"   Weight: 145 lbs

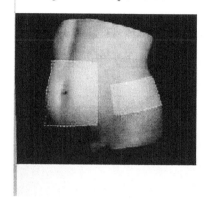

Treatment Plan

Series 1	Series 2
4 TREATMENT AREAS	4 TREATMENT AREAS
· Lower Abdomen	· Lower Abdomen
· Upper Abdomen	· Upper Abdomen
· Left Flank	· Left Flank
· Right Flank	· Right Flank
100 minutes	100 minutes

BODY TYPE B THREE FEMALE

Body Type B3
Female
Height: 5'3"   Weight: 151 lbs

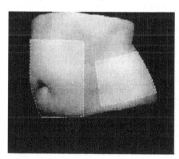

Treatment Plan

Series 1	Series 2	Series 3 (Subject to Physio)
6 TREATMENT AREAS	6 TREATMENT AREAS	6 TREATMENT AREAS
· Lower Abdomen	· Lower Abdomen	· Lower Abdomen
· Middle Abdomen	· Middle Abdomen	· Middle Abdomen
· Upper Abdomen	· Upper Abdomen	· Upper Abdomen
· Lower Left Flank	· Lower Left Flank	· Lower Left Flank
· Lower Right Flank	· Lower Right Flank	· Lower Right Flank
· Upper Left & Right Flanks	· Upper Left & Right Flanks	· Upper Left & Right Flanks
150 minutes	150 minutes	150 minutes

65

BODY TYPE C ONE FEMALE

Body Type C1
Female
Height: 5'0"   Weight: 147 lbs

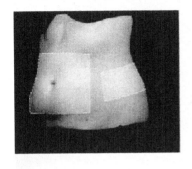

Treatment Plan

Series 1	Series 2
3 TREATMENT AREAS	3 TREATMENT AREAS
• Lower Abdomen	• Lower Abdomen
• Upper Abdomen	• Upper Abdomen
• Left & Right Flanks	• Left & Right Flanks
75 minutes	75 minutes

BODY TYPE C TWO FEMALE

Body Type C2
Female
Height: 5'6"   Weight: 192 lbs

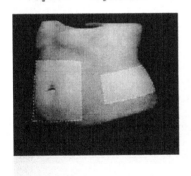

Treatment Plan

Series 1	Series 2
4 TREATMENT AREAS	4 TREATMENT AREAS
• Lower Abdomen	• Lower Abdomen
• Upper Abdomen	• Upper Abdomen
• Left Flank	• Left Flank
• Right Flank	• Right Flank
100 minutes	100 minutes

BODY TYPE C THREE FEMALE

Body Type C3
Female
Height: 5'8"   Weight: 180 lbs

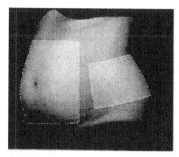

Treatment Plan

Series 1	Series 2	Series 3 (Subject to Patient)
8 TREATMENT AREAS	6 TREATMENT AREAS	6 TREATMENT AREAS
• Lower Abdomen	• Lower Abdomen	• Lower Abdomen
• Middle Abdomen	• Middle Abdomen	• Middle Abdomen
• Upper Abdomen	• Upper Abdomen	• Upper Abdomen
• Lower Left Flank	• Lower Left Flank	• Lower Left Flank
• Lower Right Flank	• Lower Right Flank	• Lower Right Flank
• Upper Left & Right Flanks	• Upper Left & Right Flanks	• Upper Left & Right Flanks
150 minutes	150 minutes	150 minutes

BODY TYPE A THREE MALE

Body Type A3
Male
Height: 5'6"   Weight: 182 lbs

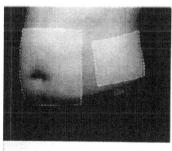

Treatment Plan

Series 1	Series 2	Series 3 (Subject to Patient)
6 TREATMENT AREAS	6 TREATMENT AREAS	6 TREATMENT AREAS
• Lower Abdomen	• Lower Abdomen	• Lower Abdomen
• Middle Abdomen	• Middle Abdomen	• Middle Abdomen
• Upper Abdomen	• Upper Abdomen	• Upper Abdomen
• Lower Left Flank	• Lower Left Flank	• Lower Left Flank
• Lower Right Flank	• Lower Right Flank	• Lower Right Flank
• Upper Left & Right Flanks	• Upper Left & Right Flanks	• Upper Left & Right Flanks
150 minutes	150 minutes	150 minutes

BODY TYPE B ONE MALE

Body Type B1
Male
Height: 5'11"   Weight: 181 lbs

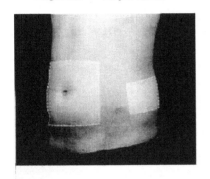

Treatment Plan

Series 1	Series 2
3 TREATMENT AREAS	3 TREATMENT AREAS
• Lower Abdomen	• Lower Abdomen
• Upper Abdomen	• Upper Abdomen
• Left & Right Flanks	• Left & Right Flanks
75 minutes	75 minutes

BODY TYPE B TWO MALE

Body Type B2
Male
Height: 5'10"   Weight: 193 lbs

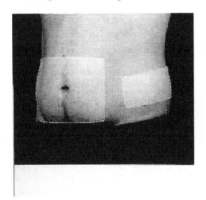

Treatment Plan

Series 1	Series 2
4 TREATMENT AREAS	4 TREATMENT AREAS
• Lower Abdomen	• Lower Abdomen
• Upper Abdomen	• Upper Abdomen
• Left Flank	• Left Flank
• Right Flank	• Right Flank
100 minutes	100 minutes

68

BODY TYPE B THREE MALE

Body Type B3
Male

Height: 5'9"   Weight: 210 lbs

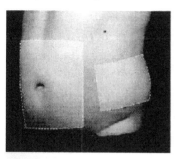

Treatment Plan

Series 1	Series 2	Series 3 (Subject to Patient)
8 TREATMENT AREAS	8 TREATMENT AREAS	8 TREATMENT AREAS
• Lower Abdomen	• Lower Abdomen	• Lower Abdomen
• Middle Abdomen	• Middle Abdomen	• Middle Abdomen
• Upper Abdomen	• Upper Abdomen	• Upper Abdomen
• Lower Left Flank	• Lower Left Flank	• Lower Left Flank
• Lower Right Flank	• Lower Right Flank	• Lower Right Flank
• Upper Left & Right Flanks	• Upper Left & Right Flanks	• Upper Left & Right Flanks
150 minutes	**150 minutes**	**150 minutes**

BODY TYPE C ONE MALE

Body Type C1
Male

Height: 6'2"   Weight: 197 lbs

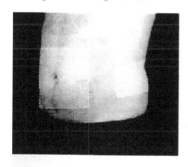

Treatment Plan

Series 1	Series 2
3 TREATMENT AREAS	3 TREATMENT AREAS
• Lower Abdomen	• Lower Abdomen
• Upper Abdomen	• Upper Abdomen
• Left & Right Flanks	• Left & Right Flanks
75 minutes	**75 minutes**

69

BODY TYPE C TWO MALE

Body Type C2
Male
Height: 6'2"   Weight: 225 lbs

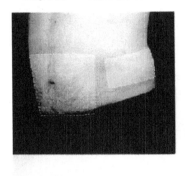

Treatment Plan

Series 1	Series 2
4 TREATMENT AREAS	4 TREATMENT AREAS
• Lower Abdomen	• Lower Abdomen
• Upper Abdomen	• Upper Abdomen
• Left Flank	• Left Flank
• Right Flank	• Right Flank
100 minutes	100 minutes

BODY TYPE C THREE MALE

Body Type C3
Male
Height: 6'2"   Weight: 228 lbs

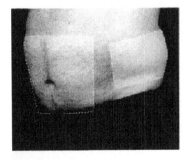

Treatment Plan

Series 1	Series 2	Series 3 (Spaced 1-2 Pohers)
6 TREATMENT AREAS	6 TREATMENT AREAS	6 TREATMENT AREAS
• Lower Abdomen	• Lower Abdomen	• Lower Abdomen
• Middle Abdomen	• Middle Abdomen	• Middle Abdomen
• Upper Abdomen	• Upper Abdomen	• Upper Abdomen
• Lower Left Flank	• Lower Left Flank	• Lower Left Flank
• Lower Right Flank	• Lower Right Flank	• Lower Right Flank
• Upper Left & Right Flanks	• Upper Left & Right Flanks	• Upper Left & Right Flanks
150 minutes	150 minutes	150 minutes

70

CHAPTER 13

Neuromodulators and Fillers

'Neuromodulator' is just another term for Botox. Botox is clostridium botulinum; it is an anaerobic gram positive bacteria commonly found in soil. It was first isolated in 1895 by Emile Van Ermengem. BT or Botox has 7 subtypes and currently only two subtypes A and B are used for cosmetics and since the B subtype has more pain associated with the injection and its duration of action is shorter, subtype A is used in most cases.

Since BT is a toxin, it can hurt you; however, the toxic dose for an average 150 pound individual would be around 3000 units or 30 vials which poses almost no risk at all. The duration of action of BT is anywhere from 3-12 months, but it is recommended to consider injections every 3-4 months so as not to allow your metabolism to completely breakdown the product and in essence having to start at the beginning again.

BT prevents the release of acetylcholine and exerts its action on the motor end plate or sympathetic nerve terminals. It prevents the muscle from contracting; which causes frowning, which causes wrinkles and fine lines.

You may have heard the names Botox, Dysport or Xeomin they are all botulinum, but made by different companies with the same goal so don't be confused by slick marketing. They all work, but the key is knowing where to place the product how much of the product to place, and whether you are even a candidate for the treatment. Perhaps the most important fact to remember is that excellent communication between yourself and your clinician will achieve the desired result you are looking for.

Botox injection is one of the most, if not the most popular non-surgical procedures performed by doctors, physician assistants, and nurses. Currently over 4 million procedures have been done.

For cosmetic purposes, Botox is ideal for the upper third of your face from the hair line to the top of the nose. The ideal areas for injection are the forehead, crow's feet around your eyes, glabella and procerus area just above the eyebrow and above the bridge of the nose. The Frontalis, Corrugator, Procerus and Orbicularis Oculi are the primary muscles injected. .

Other areas where BT is used are in cases of TMJ issues or headaches caused by muscle contraction or for hyperhidrosis or excessive sweating which may occur as your considering your treatments! Just teasing...in most cases BT injections are almost painless for a variety of reason such as very fine needles and very superficial injections along with numbing cream and or ice if necessary but in most cases it won't be necessary...easy for your clinician to say!

WHAT CAN YOU EXPECT BEFORE YOUR BT TREATMENT?

1. A review of your medical history
2. A facial analysis
3. Pre-photos
4. Review of informed consent
5. Discussion of all options and cost
6. Preparation of injection site which includes alcohol wipe of the area to reduce dead skin, decrease bacterial count
7. Placement of ice or cold compress or topical numbing cream, however if you think you need the topical anesthetic please arrive to your appointment 30 minutes early to allow the anesthetic to work.

In most cases after a consultation and treatment plan the actual treatment is completed in 5-10 minutes. There is no restriction after treatment and make up can be applied. It will normally take between 2-4 days to start and see the full effect so please be patient. We strongly suggest not to rub the area for a couple of days to allow the BT to settle in. We don't want the product to go into areas it is not intended to go. We have all seen clients with drooping eyes or fake expressions. The goal should be to look natural however everyone should have some fine lines. Our goal is to help you achieve your goals. In most cases we see the best results with a combination of BT, Fillers, and Light therapy are all used in conjunction with each other to keep your skin and face looking healthy.

The following are photos showing the most common sites of BT injections

Glabellar Lines Points of Injections   Points of Injections for Forehead Line

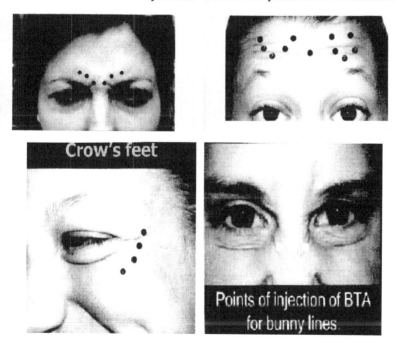

Two general options will be used when reviewing the cost of your BT treatment. We will now discuss the pros and cons of each option.

Option one - fees are based on the number of BT units used in treatment. In most cases each injection will deposit about five units of BT. Based on the consultation and your clinician, multiply the price per unit of Botox times the amount of units injected. An example would be $10/unit x 5 units=$50 per injection; therefore, 10 injections would cost $500.

Option two - fees are billed according to the area being treated. For example, the most common areas are the forehead, glabella area, and crow's feet area. Each area has a defined fee; such as $500, for example. In this case, the fee is not based on the amount of BT used, but the results necessary to achieve an acceptable outcome.

It is our opinion that the fee should be based on the expertise, knowledge, and ability of the clinician; and the ability to offer total care which meets or exceeds your expectations.

POTENTIAL COMPLICATION OF BT INJECTIONS:

1. BT injections are contraindicated in clients with neuromuscular diseases such as amyotrophic lateral sclerosis and myasthenia gravis

2. BT injections are contraindicated in clients with infection at the site of the BT injection

3. BT injections are contraindicated in pregnant clients or lactating women

4. BT injections should be avoided in clients taking aminoglycoside and or use anticholinergic drugs

SOME ADVERSE EVENTS ARE:

1. Arrhythmia

2. Headache

3. Dry eye

4. Ocular pain

5. Bruising- when bruising occurs consider concealer yellow base for blue bruising, green base for red bruising, white base for brown bruising and lavender base for yellow bruising.

6. Upper eyelid ptosis or droopy eyelid consider apraclonidine (lopidine.5% solution)

Time and patience will resolve most adverse side effects.

FILLERS

Fillers, sometimes referred as dermal fillers, were first FDA approved in 1981. Fillers were first used in the skin in Europe in 1996. In most cases they are resorbable materials of collagen, hyaluronic acid, hydroxyethyl, methacrylate, dextran, polylactic acid. All of these products will be enzymatically metabolized or phagocytized and have very little tissue reaction.

In most cases the fillers are divided into permanent and semi-permanent options. Most clinician would agree that nothing is really permanent except death and taxes however, in the aesthetic world a product that lasts over two years is generally considered permanent. Examples of these products are Silicone, Teflon and PMMA or polymethylmethacrylate. Although all products have advantages and disadvantages most clinicians will guide you toward the semi-permanent products, which are in most cases hyaluronic acid or HA. These products have proven to be very safe and effective with very little negative side effects.

HA is found normally in all humans and makes up the ground substance of the dermis, which is the lower layer of your skin. HA makes up about 56% of your skin, 28% of your connective tissue, and 8% of your muscles. HA (Hylaform) is derived from animals. It can also be derived from the bacteria streptococcus, which is the substance used in Juvederm and Restylane.

Most fillers are not radiopaque, meaning they do not show up on a radiograph; and, most fillers last between 4-12 months.In addition, most fillers are used on fine lines and wrinkle and folds. The most common areas are the cheeks, lips and nasolabial fold areas. Many times fillers have a local anesthetic incorporated with the product. After the first injection, the area will become numb--similar to a dental injection--and in most cases the client would feel little or no pain. Full result usually occurs in about 2 days, so please be patient. Your clinician may massage the filler into various areas to give the most natural results.

Most companies that manufacture fillers have different classes of products. These products have various names but in general they have different consistency. Some fillers are soft and more watery, and other are stiffer and denser and some fall somewhere in between. The clinician is trained to be aware of which products work best for the client. For example, most clients would prefer a softer feeling product for the lips and perhaps a denser product for the cheeks and something in between for the nasolabial fold area.

The goal of your clinician is to open up the communication so we deliver the right product to the right areas in the correct amount to give you the results you are looking for.

WHEN IT COMES TO COST AGAIN TWO OPTIONS ARE GENERALLY CONSIDERED:

Option One - you will be charged by the amount of filler used. In most cases but not all the fillers come in pre-packaged syringes and each syringe contains 1ml of filler. Please keep in mind we cannot use the same syringe on different clients so whether you use .5ml or the full 1.0 ml the cost will be the same. For example if each syringe is $750.00 that would be your charge or fee, whether we use it all or just some of the filler.

Option Two - you will be charged for the area; whether that is the cheeks, nasolabial fold, or lips. An example would be upper lip is

$750.00 and lower lip would be $750.00 regardless of the amount of filler used.

Each option has its advantages and disadvantages. Discuss the options with your clinician so that you fully understand the care and service you will be receiving and paying for.

What is difficult is each company or manufacturer has a different fee for each of their fillers. So even though they are all called 'fillers,' one product may cost $300.00 to purchase and another product may be $900.00.

What you should consider with your clinician is not just cost and your clinician's expertise and experience but how long is the expected duration of the filler to last! For example only if filler A is $300.00 but has to be touched up every 3 months and filler B is $900.00 but last 12 months your overall cost is much better with Filler B. In the end, we suggest that you not only consider cost, but more importantly, outcome. Consider the right product for the right location to give you the best results.

THE FOLLOWING IS A PHOTO PROVIDING YOU WILL AREA OF POSSIBLE FILLER PLACEMENT:

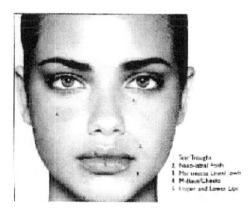

ADVERSE EFFECTS TO FILLERS:

1. Pain

2. Swelling

3. Bruising

4. Tissue breakdown

In most cases, time and patience will solve most issues. Apply warm compresses and hyaluronidase (an enzyme that breaks down HA) if too much was administered. Usually 10-75 units will reverse HA effects. In some cases antibiotics will be necessary, debridement and makeup concealers.

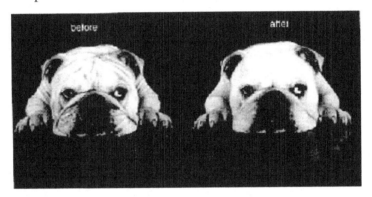

CHAPTER 14

PRP - Plasma Rich Platelets

PRP is a technique to provide faster healing with less postoperative pain and complications. With PRP we are taking your blood and spinning it down to get a high concentration of platelets along with various blood products such as:

1. PDGF or platelet derived growth factor

2. TGF or transforming growth factor

3. VEGF or vascular endothelial growth factor

4. IGF or insulin like growth factor

5. ECM or extracellular matrix

It is the high concentration of these growth factors that have proven to be beneficial in some many areas of medicine and healthcare. The following are just a few of the areas PRP is being used:

1. Problematic wound healing

2. Bone defects

3. Cosmetic and gastrointestinal surgeries and skin rejuvenation

The topical or injected PRP appears to help stimulate facial skin by improving its appearance by inducing new collagen synthesis. PRP injected into the scalp also seems to significantly help in female and male pattern baldness, but at present time it seems to benefit females more.

In most cases, your clinician will take several vials of your blood. That blood will get spun down in a centrifuge at 7000 rpms for about 13-15 minutes. Your clinician will take the upper layer and spin that down at 3000 rpms for about 4-5 minutes; then, he/she will take that upper layer and apply it to your skin or scalp area to jump start your treatment.

The PRP treatment is additional advanced care in clients who need additional care and treatment in order to get the best results.

However, results can vary from client to client due to the inconsistent potency and concentration of PRP.

CHAPTER 15

Kybella and PDO Threads

Kybella is a non-surgical injectable technique that focuses on the submental area, or that area under the chin. It consists of a series of injections of a chemical called deoxycholic acid. Deoxycholic acid targets fat cells in the area of the injection and kills those cells. No incisions are required and down time is minimal in most cases. The ideal candidate is over the age of 18 with moderate to severe fat beneath the chin. Surveys by the American Society for Dermatologic Surgery have found about 67% of individuals are bothered by excess fat under the chin or neck area. Currently Kybella is the only injectable treatment approved by the FDA to treat the appearance of a double chin.

Deoxycholic acid is a bile acid that is naturally produced by your body to help absorb fat. Kybella injections use a synthetic form of this acid. After the injection, the acid destroys fat cells beneath the chin area so it cannot store anymore fat. It is important to understand deoxycholic acid can kill other cells also, and this why you must have a consultation with your clinician about all risk and benefits.

Prior to treatment a complete review of your health history must be done. You must inform your clinician of any difficulties swallowing or bleeding issues. We advise you to avoid treatment if you're pregnant or lactating. It is suggested you also avoid treatment if you're planning on any head and neck surgeries in the near future. Your face will be thoroughly washed and cleaned to decrease any chance of infection, and it is strongly advised you avoid ibuprofen and acetaminophen, which increases the chance of bruising--which can and does occur frequently.

Your clinician will mark the injection sites under your chin and in most cases you can expect between 20-50 injections under your chin area. Prior to the injections a topical numbing cream or ice pack will minimize any discomfort. You can expect to see changes over the next few weeks. Many times this is a good alternative to surgical procedures such as liposuction. In many cases only one treatment will be necessary, but in some case as many as six treatments may be necessary to get the acquired results. It is suggested each appointment be scheduled about 4 weeks apart.

Several studies stated about 82% of the individuals reported significant improvement in the submental region for fat reduction.

PDO THREADS

PDO therapy is a cosmetic technique that lifts and tightens sagging skin tissues by inducing collagen production. PDO stands for polydioxanone threads which are similar to medical sutures. The threads are resorbable and can be used almost anywhere however in most cases are used to lift loose skin on the face and neck with minimal downtime.

As we age the effects of gravity start to set in and become more noticeable on our faces. Facial support structure weakens as we lose facial fat. This becomes increasingly noticeable around the eyebrows and around the eyes in general along with cheeks and jowls and neck area. Our face starts to look longer and more square-shaped and older looking. Prior to considering a face lift this procedure and technique may be right for you.

PDO threads are and option to achieve natural results with no surgery and very little discomfort. Most procedures can be completed in an hour (or at a lunch time!) and is an exceptional option for the neck and jawline.

A beautiful face which is healthy has a general V shape. Although Botox and filler can be placed almost anywhere in the lower third of the face those treatments can be more challenging, and PDO threads may be the best option.

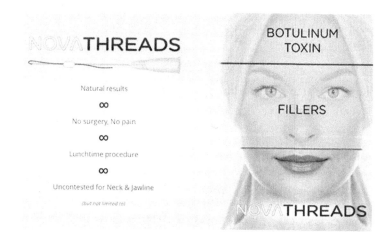

NOVATHREADS

Natural results

∞

No surgery, No pain

∞

Lunchtime procedure

∞

Uncontested for Neck & Jawline

(but not limited to)

BOTULINUM TOXIN

FILLERS

NOVATHREADS

PDO threads are FDA approved and are fully absorbed within 4-6 months without leaving any scars. The sutures create an inflammatory response with your skin, and as the skin repairs new collagen is formed. The new skin will heal itself creating a younger and healthier look.

The ideal client shows minimal signs of aging and needs just a small lift. Other candidates include clients who have had some relapse from a previous plastic surgery or those clients who do not wish to undergo a surgical facelift or neck lift.

THE STEPS INVOLVED WHEN PERFORMING A PDO THREAD LIFT:

1. Review of medical history
2. The site area cleaned with alcohol
3. Numbing topical cream placed on treatment area
4. The injection spots are labeled
5. The threads are then inserted under the skin in precise locations using a small hollow needle to lift and support the droopy elements without removing any skin. The inserted thread is then able to grasp onto droopy skin and soft tissue to reposition the skin. No cuts or incisions are made.
6. When the lift is secured the hollow needle is removed without leaving any scars

7. Depending on desired effect will determine how many sutures will be used.

There are several types of threads and different techniques. In most cases the threads are either smooth or barbed. It will be up to you and your clinician to determine the best technique to reach your ideal outcome.

In general terms, the barbed type of threads may provide a more dramatic and long-lasting result, while the smooth thread will produce a more natural and gradual result.

In most cases OTC Tylenol and or Advil will be all that is needed. You can expect mild swelling and bruising for a few days. It is suggested you place ice on the area as well as arnica for the first few days while avoiding strenuous activity

Although results are immediate, they become more noticeable a few weeks post treatment.

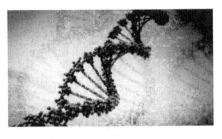

∞ In medical terms **"Selective Inflammatory Response"** it is the principle behind a lot of aesthetic procedures (such as Fractional Laser, Chemical Peels & MicroNeedling). Our skin is very good at repairing itself, and by inserting the THREADS we make it "heal" itself by creating new collagen, naturally!

YOUR SKIN GENTLY REACTS TO THE INSERTED THREADS

∞ Yes, PDO is fully absorbable, but that doesn't mean your skin won't react to it. During the 4 to 6 months needed to fully absorb the PDO suture, your skin is also repairing itself around it.

∞ It's "controlled healing" happening underneath the skin!

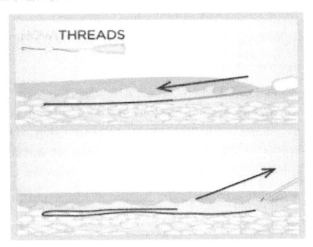

CHAPTER 16

Skin Products

You have invested time and money to make yourself look and feel great! Now it is time to invest in home care products to be used correctly every day to keep you looking young and feeling great. Remember skin care and skin care products are not just for women. We see more and more men that understand that it's not only important to keep your body in shape, but keeping your skin in shape and healthy is just as important.

What you should be looking for in any skin care product is the following… A product line that has extensive research, innovation, and education behind each and every product. The products should focus on preventive measures, protective measures, and corrective measures. The three critical areas of prevent, protect, and correct should be available for the face, body, neck chest and hand regions. Since we know almost everyone is under hydrated the product line should offer moisturizers.

In order for any product to work correctly and be truly effective should be pure, formulated at a correct pH and be of the correct concentration.

Step one will always be to cleanse and tone, to lift impurities and oils off the skin, to exfoliate dead skin cells away, and to balance your pH levels. For most of us the ideal pH of your skin should be between 4.0- 5.5.

Step two is to prevent damage or oxidation reactions to your skin. This is accomplished by the use of antioxidant protection from environmental skin damage. Remember that sunscreens are an essential first line of defense but only block about 55% of damaging free radicals that cause chemical reaction in the skin that can be harmful. Your products should provide advanced protection against UV, infrared radiation A and pollution induced aging and skin damage.

Step three, your products should correct and address specific skin concerns. Since over time skin changes and signs of aging will occur. These changes will be fine lines, wrinkles, discoloration, and loss of elasticity. These changes can be the result of collagen breakdown along with slower cell turnover and loss of moisture. Your products should promote reparative, brightening, and exfoliating ingredients to help you obtain a healthier skin and more youthful appearance. Remember your skin's ability to self-repair will decline by more than 50% by middle age.

Step four moisturizing will help prevent moisture loss and improve skin smoothness. These products should have multi-functional ingredients that nourish, protect and exfoliate as they hydrate the skin and restore its elasticity. Products that use hyaluronic acid hold up to 1000x its weight in water.

Step five is protection, which is the first line of defense against premature aging and skin cancer. These products should have mineral and chemical sunscreen filters to provide broad spectrum of UVA/UVB protection. Newer products should contain Z-Cote which is a transparent mineral zinc oxide to physically protect skin from damaging UVA rays, which are responsible for aging, and UVB rays which are responsible for burning. Remember UVA rays can penetrate through clouds and glass and account for 95% of the UV radiation reaching the earth's surface.

You should consider a skincare system that is comprehensive and designed to effectively address specific skin concerns and feature cleanser, toners, antioxidants, moisturizing and corrective products along with sunscreens to meet your needs and keep your skin young looking and feeling great -- while addressing discolorations, signs of aging, acne, uneven skin tones and sensitive skin types.

CHAPTER 17

Makeup

The primary of goal of makeup is to enhance your natural beauty by bringing out the most attractive features of the face while minimizing those less attractive features. In most cases a blend of makeup artistry, hairstyle and clothing choices will provide the best results along with a confident attitude good posture and an overall feeling of being pleased with yourself inside and out.

When considering color you should understand that Hue is the actual color we see and is the distinct characteristic of the color. Tint is when white is added to a pure hue. Shade is adding black to a pure hue. Tone is adding gray to a pure hue. Saturation is the intensity or strength of a color making it either pale or strong. Value is the brightness of a color or how light or dark it is.

Remember warm colors have a yellow undertone while cool colors have a blue undertone. Red and Greens can be both cool and warm.

Makeup like other things can be inexpensive, or very expensive, and in most cases you get what you pay for. Look at your products carefully. Remember most products come in many forms such as powders, creams and liquids.

Foundation is also known as base makeup and is used to even out skin tone and color while concealing imperfections and protecting your skin from the outside elements of climate, dirt, and pollutions. Remember foundation can improve dark circles, blemishes pigmentation redness along with many other imperfections. In general you will most likely consider darker colors in the summer and lighter colors in the winter. Water-based foundation provides a more matte finish and are many times best for oily skin types. Your foundation should always be matched as closely as possible to actual skin tone.

Concealers are used to cover up discolorations and may be applied before or after your foundation. Concealers are available in pots, pencils, wands or sticks along with a variety of colors and can contain moisturizer or control oil depending on the concealer formulation. Remember concealers should be one to two shades lighter than your foundation.

Face powder is used to add a matte or non-shiny finish to your face. It should enhance the skin's natural color and is used to set your foundation. Powder generally comes in two forms, loose, or pressed. They also come in a variety of tints, shades and different weights -- referred to as sheer to heavy. You should always apply powder with a brush and it should match the natural skin tone and work well with foundation.

Blush will give your face a natural looking glow and help create facial contours. It should be applied with a brush just below the cheekbones.

Eye shadow accentuates and contours the eye, which in most cases is the focal point in makeup design. They come in almost all colors and finishes such as matte, frost and shimmer.

Eye liner is also used to emphasize the eyes. With eyeliner you can create a line on the eyelid close to the lashes to make the eyes appear larger and lashes fuller.

Eyebrow color helps frame your eyes by creating the correct shape that enhances your face.

Mascara darkens and defines and thickens the eyelashes.

Lip color is ideal to define and bring attention to your lips.

Eye makeup remover is either oil based or water based. Oil based usually is mineral oil and water based are usually witch hazel based.

Proper supplies and equipment are important for best results. That means you need the correct brushes for powder, blush, concealer, eyeshadow, eyeliner, lash and brow and lip brush to get the best out of your products and provide the best and most consistent results. Along with brushes you should also have sponges for blending, lash curler and comb and wand to use for your mascara.

WHEN YOU SELECT MAKEUP COLORS REMEMBER THE THREE MOST IMPORTANT THINGS.

1. Skin color
2. Eye color
3. Hair color

When deciding on skin color, choices are light, medium, or dark When choosing eye colors remember complementary colors for blue eyes are orange shades. For green eyes, consider red as the complementary color. Brown eyes are considered neutral so almost any color can work.

Remember that makeup is one area in aesthetics where you have to apply in a downward fashion going with the direction of the vellus hairs on the face.

UNDERSTAND THAT THE HUMAN FACE COMES IN MANY SHADES BUT FOR MOST THERE WILL BE A DOMINANT SHAPE SUCH AS:

- Oval
- Round
- Square
- Rectangle of oblong
- Triangle or pear shape
- Heart
- Diamond

It makes sense to understand facial type to choose corrective makeup techniques to get the best results. The following are some tricks of the trade to get you the look you're after.

For small face and short thick neck you should consider slightly darker foundation on the side of neck than the one used on the face. This will make the neck appear thinner and longer.

If your face is to round and your looking to soften it up or square it up, consider using two foundations a light and a dark with the darker shade blended on the outer edges of the temples cheekbones and jawline and lighter foundation from the center of the forehead down to center of the face to the tip of the chin.

If your face is too triangular apply a darker foundation over the chin and neck and a lighter foundation through the cheeks and under the eyes to temples and toward the forehead and then blend them together over the forehead for a smooth and natural finish.

If your face is too narrow, blend a light shade of foundation over the outer edges of the cheekbones to bring out the sides of the face.

If your jaw is too wide consider applying a darker foundation below the cheekbones and along the jawline and blend into the neck.

If you have double chin consider applying shading under the jawline and chin over the full area.

If you have a long heavy chin consider applying darker foundation over the area.

If you have a receding chin consider using a lighter foundation than the one used on the face.

If you have a protruding forehead apply a darker shade of foundation over the forehead area.

If you have a narrow forehead apply a lighter foundation along the hairline and blend onto the forehead.

If you have a wide nose apply foundation a shade lighter to the center of the nose and apply darker foundation on both sides of the nose and blend them together.

If you have a short nose apply a lighter shade of foundation blended onto the tip of the nose and between the eyes.

These techniques can be applied to the eyes and lips. Let our clinicians guide you through all the endless techniques to help you achieve your non-surgical goals.

In order to continue to recruit, convert, and retain clients we must constantly provide information and concern for your non-surgical esthetic needs. We must inform you about all options and risks. We must help you decide on treatments and help you in our assessment of what is needed. We have to constantly provide up-to-date communication and education to provide you with the knowledge to make an informed decision. We need to set realistic expectations for your care and treatment.

Our goal is to establish what we call BLT or what we hope to obtain is you Believe us, Like us, and Trust us.

We hope this guide will help you make the most informed consent to achieve your non-surgical esthetic goals. We are committed to providing you with the highest level of care and service, and we hope you can sense our dedication to that process by reading this informative publication.

THANK YOU

Appendix and Resources

Milady Standard Fundamentals Esthetics, authors Joel Gerson, Janet D'Angelo, Sallie Deitz, Shelly Lotz, Eleventh Edition, Cengage Learning, Chapters 3,4,18 and 20

Invisible, authors Sidney Kina and August Bruguera, ISBN 978-85-367-0085-4, Publishing Director Milton Hecht copyright 2008, Chapter 1 and 2

To both the Cynosure and Cutera companies for providing education training and knowledge to clinicians to improve the care and treatment of are most important assets: our clients.

To Jolie Health and Beauty School for my education and training in the field of aesthetics and a special thanks to Ms. Jean, Ms. Sandy, Ms. Amanda and Ms. Christina for your patience in teaching me the importance of proper skin care.

To National Laser Institute for continuing to offer education and knowledge to help us understand the exceptional field of medical and laser cosmetics

To the many dedicated Dermatologist, Plastic Surgeons who have provided time and expertise in teaching me and so many others how to improve one's appearance with non-surgical options, but the expertise to understand what can and cannot be done.

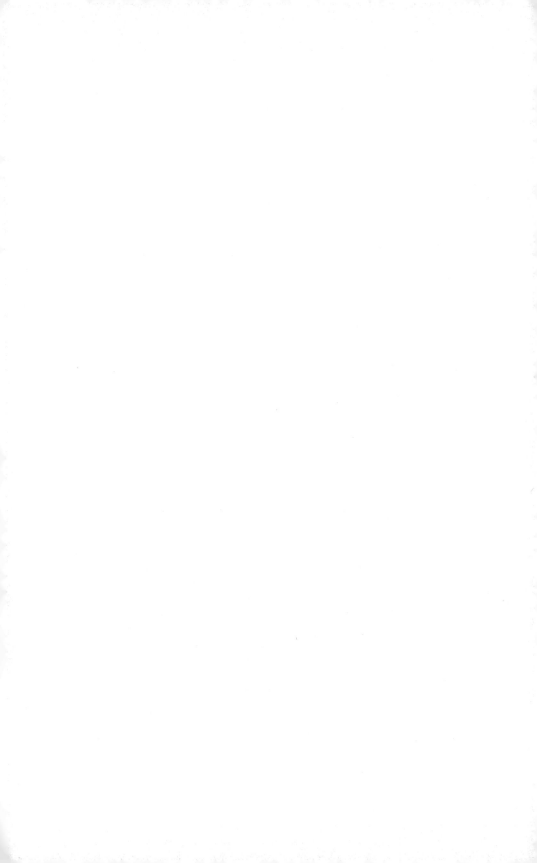

Made in the
USA
Middletown, DE